T0113809

JOURNEY TO ACCEPTANCE

SPIRITUAL RELEASE FROM FOOD BONDAGE

DONNA FRIEND

WESTBOW
PRESS®
A DIVISION OF THOMAS NELSON
& ZONDERVAN

Scripture quotations taken from the Holy Bible, New Living Translation,
Copyright © 1996, 2004. Used by permission of Tyndale House
Publishers, Inc., Wheaton, Illinois 60189. All rights reserved.

Scripture quotations are from The Holy Bible, English Standard Version®
(ESV®), copyright © 2001 by Crossway, a publishing ministry of Good
News Publishers. Used by permission. All rights reserved.
Scripture taken from the Amplified Bible, copyright © 1954, 1958, 1962,
1964, 1965, 1987 by The Lockman Foundation. Used by permission.

Scripture taken from the American Standard Version of the Bible.

WestBow Press books may be ordered through booksellers or by contacting:

WestBow Press
A Division of Thomas Nelson & Zondervan
1663 Liberty Drive
Bloomington, IN 47403
www.westbowpress.com
1 (866) 928-1240

ISBN: 978-1-5127-3857-5 (sc)
ISBN: 978-1-5127-3856-8 (e)

Print information available on the last page.

WestBow Press rev. date: 04/25/2016

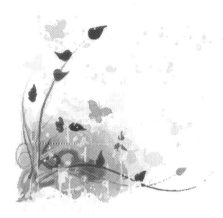

Dedications

This is yet another book in the Christian world inspired by the Holy Spirit's urging to share with others what He has accomplished in a fellow believer's life. I thank God for writing every word on each page and walking me through this valuable lesson of being set free from food bondage. I thank my husband, Eric, for all of his love, support, and encouragement as I worked on this project during the last 4 years of his life. I know you are smiling from heaven. A big thank you to my children, Rob and Allie, for allowing me the space and time to see this project through to completion. A special thank you goes out to Eileen Atwood for being the catalyst for publishing. Thank you to my friends and family for being my biggest cheerleaders!

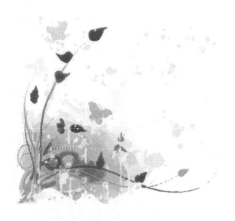

Foreward

In the Gospel of John, Chapter 8 and verse 36 we are given this simple, yet wonderful assurance by Jesus:

"So if the Son sets you free, you are truly free."

And He should know, because he is the Son of God who sets us free!

In fact, Jesus had said just a few verses earlier (8:32):

"And you will know the truth, and the truth will set you free."

And He should certainly know about that as well, shouldn't He?

Because, after all, He IS the Way, the Truth, and the Life! (John 14:6)

All of this Biblical truth raises an interesting question/dilemma -

"If we've been set free, then why do we often still feel trapped in bondage to our old habits?"

The Apostle Paul posed a similar question to the believers in the church at Colossae:

"You have died with Christ, and he has set you free from the spiritual powers of this world. So why do you keep on following the rules of the world, such as, ²¹ "Don't handle! Don't taste! Don't touch!"? ²² Such rules are mere human teachings about things that deteriorate as we use them. ²³ These rules may seem wise because they require strong devotion, pious self-denial, and severe bodily discipline. But they provide no help in conquering a person's evil desires." (Colossians 2:20-23)

In the end, there is only one real answer. The prophet Hosea expressed it in describing God's sorrow at our human condition in Hosea 4:6

"My people are being destroyed because they don't know me."

Thankfully, *"being destroyed"* doesn't have to be the case in our lives.

Author and Christian Counselor Donna Friend has blessed us with this insightful instruction manual, firmly rooted in scripture and drawing upon her years of dedicated training and ministry experience. Within these pages she provides a framework for freedom based upon the crucial understanding that it's never enough to know about God – Our freedom comes from truly knowing God, and knowing who God made us to be.

In this valuable book Donna addresses a series of key topics, including:

- The voices that influence our self-perception

- Inner Vows
- The essential nature of forgiveness
- Dangerous emotions
- Why worrying is a trap
- And many more "freeing" strategies

Starting with a solid Biblical foundation, Donna is able to provide additional encouragement through personal testimonies of those who have been truly set free by coming to know who they are in Jesus Christ.

Most importantly, Donna has provided a series of dynamic, powerful prayers that can be implemented at each step along the journey to freedom.

I thank God for the privilege of knowing Donna and seeing the impact of her ministry in the lives of so many individuals. I know that this book is God's way of allowing her to reach, and to help, more people than ever.

May you, dear reader, be blessed beyond measure by the words and the truth you are about to encounter.

Sincerely,

Pastor Steve Rahter
Praise Tabernacle

Contents

Dedications v
Foreward vii
Acknowledgement xiii
Introduction xv

Chapter 1   The Voices 1
Chapter 2   Emotions 9
Chapter 3   Inner Vows 26
Chapter 4   Do Not Worry 38
Chapter 5   Gluttony 50
Chapter 6   Perfectionism 60
Chapter 7   Lust of the flesh, Lust of the eyes,
            Pride of life and Jonah revisited 71

Afterword 79
Bibliography (Works Cited) 81

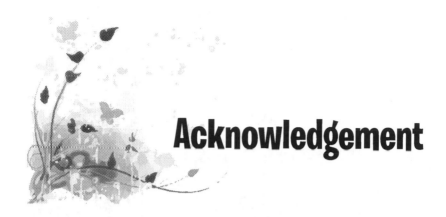

Acknowledgement

A big *thank you* goes out to Pastor Steve Rahter, Karen Oliver and Maria Castillo for assisting this first time writer in editing. I couldn't have finished this project without all of your love and guidance. May God richly bless each of you!

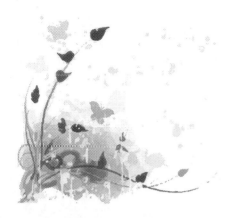

Introduction

"Have you heard the latest on saturated fat?" "What's your BMI?" "What is your carb to protein ratio for your size and weight?" Everyday there are questions and comments swirling around about our food intake. The medical world is constantly offering new opinions and there are many people who coined themselves experts when it comes to eating, dieting and weight loss. But what does God say about all the hype? How do you know when you have crossed the line over into food bondage?

This book was inspired by my many years of struggling through all of the above questions and so many more. Because we need food in order to survive, nourishing our bodies can quickly turn into a stumbling block for many people. Christians are not an exception to this rule. In fact, it seems to be the often unspoken sin in the Body of Christ.

As you take the journey through the chapters of this book, my prayer is that every chain of food bondage that is holding you down will be broken in Jesus' name.

I sincerely ask you to work diligently on each chapter with the Lord. This book is not a race to the finish. The chapters are designed to tear down the strongholds in your life that have held you down in food bondage.

I urge you to linger over the prayer at the end of each chapter. There is an anointing that abides in each prayer to set you free. May this book be your final journey in your struggle with food and I pray your soul will be at peace as you finish the last chapter!

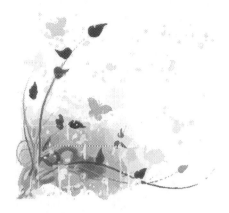

Chapter 1
The Voices

I have little doubt you have opened this book hoping and praying that it will be the last input you will ever need on being free from the bondage of weight control. I pray that it will be the key that unlocks the door to all God wants to do for you in this area of your life.

Some of you may be asking yourselves, "What is this bondage and how did I get here in the first place?" The definition of bondage is to be *in slavery or involuntary servitude.* You are not meant to live in bondage to any earthly things. You most likely got to this place because you shut the door on too many spiritual closets that need to be cleaned out. This book is designed to uproot and tear down spiritual strongholds that compel you to overeat. God wants to deal with these issues, so you can walk in freedom. I don't want you to feel like it's a formula of some sort, but as believers, we have been given the keys to the Kingdom of heaven as it states in Matthew.

Matthew 18:18 (ASV) " Verily I say unto you, what things soever ye shall bind on earth shall be bound in heaven; and what things soever ye shall loose on earth shall be loosed in heaven."

You possess the power to bind and loose, to uproot the hidden things, and slam the door shut on the enemy. It is necessary to take God as your partner and work as a team.

Sometimes, as a believer, you expect God to do everything for you. If He did, how would you ever learn from your mistakes. As a child of heaven, it's your responsibility to go to God first regarding the spiritual aspect of illness, addiction, bondages and everything else that is interfering with your life. You can't rely on the world's methodology as your first line of attack. You need to pull on the Kingdom of heaven first. God cares about the things that concern you. He wants to partner with you in all of your successes, even eating.

As you begin your journey, you must *draw a line in the sand* with yourself.

What does that really mean? One definition explains it as such, *"A point (physical, decisional, etc.) beyond which one will proceed no further."* The second meaning is, *"That of a point beyond which, once the decision to go beyond it is made, the decision and its resulting consequences are permanently decided and irreversible."* I want this decision for you to be so permanent in your life that you will never look back!

Jesus drew in the sand in John chapter 8 when the Scribes and Pharisees were accusing the woman caught in adultery. It may or may not have been a line He was drawing, but He was defining a new boundary.

John 8:3-11 (ASV) 3 "And the Scribes and the Pharisees bring a woman taken in adultery; and having set her in the midst, 4 they say unto him, Teacher, this woman hath been taken in adultery, in the very act. 5 Now in the law Moses commanded us to stone such: what then sayest thou of her? 6 And this they said, trying him, that they might have whereof to accuse him. But Jesus stooped down, and with his finger wrote on the ground. 7 But when they continued asking him, he lifted up himself, and said unto them, He that is without sin among you, let him first cast a stone at her. 8 And again he stooped down, and with his finger wrote on the ground. 9 And they, when they heard it, went out one by one, beginning from the eldest, even unto the last: and Jesus was left alone, and the woman, where she was, in the midst. 10 And Jesus lifted up himself, and said unto her, Woman, where are they? did no man condemn thee? 11 And she said, No man, Lord. And Jesus said, Neither do I condemn thee: go thy way; from henceforth sin no more."

This is your starting point to *draw a line in the sand* with yourself and *go and sin no more*. Part of that new journey is quieting the voices in your mind. God did not condemn her, He told her to stop doing what she was doing.

How do you quiet the voices in your mind? Jonah's little whale adventure is a great example of this concept. He was commissioned to warn the populace of Nineveh of the coming judgement. One of the voices in his mind was the fear of how the people of Nineveh would respond to him. That voice is *fear of man*. Fear of man means that you are more concerned with what others think of you than what God thinks of you. How about the voices in our world that tell you how to look, what to wear and how gracefully you should be aging. When you believe you have to meet this standard it's a form of idolatry and fear of man.

As you know, the Lord caused a whale to swallow Jonah, where he stayed in it's belly for 3 days and 3 nights. Jonah couldn't hear outside input and I bet there was no *fear of man* in the whale. I also bet that Jonah wasn't wondering if his hips looked big in his tunic while he sat in that putrid smell wondering if he would ever see daylight again. I am sure he wasn't thinking about how flat his stomach would look when he had gone 3 days or more without eating.

His only concern was survival and coming to a place of true repentance before his God.

As Jonah sat in that whale, his concern for Nineveh's response to him became secondary to hearing what God had to say. It is the same for you. You need to starve the voices that have overtaken your mind. One of the definitions of the word *starve* is to cause something to die from lack of feeding it. Starve *fear of man*; starve *self-condemnation*; starve what you have allowed the world to heap on top of you. You need to stop hating self and come into agreement with how Father God sees you. He sees you perfected through the blood of Jesus.

You can't serve two masters. You will love one and hate the other. Jesus explains this in the gospel of Matthew.

Matthew 6:24(ASV) "No one can serve two masters; for either he will hate the one and love the other, or he will stand by and be devoted to the one and despise and be against the other. You cannot serve God and mammon."

Many people only apply this scripture to money and possessions, however, the very next verse speaks of food, the body and clothing and not to be so focused on all of it.

Matthew 6:25 (ASV) "That is why I tell you not to worry about everyday life-whether you have enough food and drink, or enough clothes to wear. Isn't life more than food, and your body more than clothing?"

You serve yourself when you agree with the world that you need to fit into a size 2 if you are really a size 4,6,8, 10, 12 and so on. You begin to resist what is real. The definition of resist is *trying to prevent something by action or argument.* You begin to dismiss reality as you try to fit into the world's mold. You will try every diet, hop on board with every fad. Most of you have even tried things (pills, powders, liquid diets) even if you know it could harm your body. All of these expensive, over-inflated gimmicks attempted for the sake of quieting the voices in your head that tell you how to get to that elusive size 2. Your day and your thoughts are consumed with getting there and you've convinced yourself that this is a healthy goal.

Just like you, I am speaking from personal experience. Most of my childhood years were spent living on a farm. When I was a little girl, I was very aware (by 7 or 8 years old) that I was heavier than the other girls. By the time I was nine or ten, I was dieting. I could muster enough willpower to last a day or two and then would fall off the preverbal horse and go right back to self-medicating with food, in total defeat!

By the time I was in seventh grade, I was focused on my weight most of the time. Most of my friends were skinny and they didn't ever have to think about what they ate. By this time in my life, I had a new motivation for getting thin…boys. My need for approval from the opposite sex was intense. I had empty places that needed filling and I thought attention from guys was the answer. In order to get that attention, I needed to not be fat. I hated exercise, period! I was not gifted in the athletic department so I avoided physical activity. My

Mother was a great cook and also loved to bake. There was dessert at my house every night. Half of my family could eat whatever they wanted, while the other half of us struggled constantly with our size.

Puberty made a huge difference for me and most of my weight fell off, however, at that point I was so focused on perfection of body and being skinny instead of healthy, that I never laid down my constant need to be smaller. The scale was my friend and my adversary at the same time (sometimes even on the same day.)

I was trying to serve two gods. I lived that way for decades. Are you currently serving two gods? Every day that you get on the scale and it's not where you want to be, another layer of self-disappointment creeps in. Perhaps another layer of feeling like you are a failure.

What does this do to your spirit? It leaves you double-minded about who you are. In order to go forward you need to get before the Lord and ask for forgiveness for serving two masters. You have come into agreement with those voices of *self-condemnation* and *fear of man*. It is necessary to break off the agreement you made in order to move ahead. Please pray this prayer and seek Jesus.

Dear Heavenly Father,

I thank you that I have access to the throne of grace through the Blood of Jesus. I come to you with a repentant heart. I confess my sins of *self-condemnation* and *fear of man*. I ask you to forgive me for trying to serve two masters. I confess the specific sins of _____(name the things the the Holy Spirit has been showing you as you have read this chapter e.g., the scale, size issues, worrying about what others think) I sit before You quietly and ask You to bring to my remembrance any other areas that I may have missed (as He brings them, ask for forgiveness.) I break every agreement I have made with the world's standards for my appearance and come into agreement with You and what You have to say about my weight, my body image and my eating and exercise habits. I thank you that You will show me all things that I need to do to treat my body as a temple for the Holy Spirit. In Jesus name I pray, Amen.

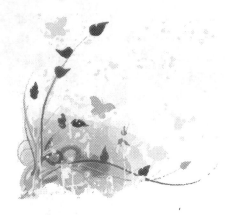

Notes

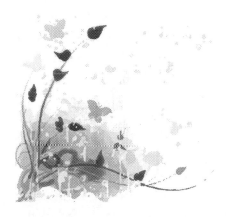

Chapter 2
Emotions

Emotions are such an amazing part of your God-given makeup. They can be your best friend or your worst enemy. Unless you are apathetic, most of you express emotion from the moment you wake up until you close your eyes to sleep. The emotions you will explore in this chapter are very characteristic of weight gain.

These emotions, in particular, cause people to carry extra weight as a shield of protection to guard themselves from pain. Excess weight can be worn like protective clothing to shut potentially hurtful people out.

Let's explore the following:

1. Self-pity - The Oxford English Dictionary describes this as, *excessive concern with and unhappiness over one's own troubles.* You may have some feelings of regret or sorrow over events and people that have hurt you. You focus on self and the wrongs that have been done to you. You may also be focused daily on what is going wrong instead of what is good and right

in your life. Perhaps you had role models in your life that modeled negative, self-absorbed behavior.

As a counselor, I can tell you that self-pity can be a serious stronghold in a person's life. It can lock you into a position of not seeing your blame in a situation or being able to take responsibility for your actions. Self-pity says, "This is all your fault, not mine." or "My life will never be good again because of what you did to me!" One of my favorite speakers a few decades ago use to say, "Aren't you just so tired of forty year old whining people who are still blaming their whole lives on their parents?" There comes a point in all of our lives when we must stop feeling sorry for ourselves and our circumstances and take responsibility for where we are and how we stand in our relationships with others. Self-pity is also very much connected to the second emotion which is:

2. Self-righteousness - The term self-righteous is defined by www.yourdictionary.com as, *filled with or showing a conviction of being morally superior, or more righteous than others; smugly virtuous.* Maybe you have fallen into a pattern of assuming that you have the right to see the sin in others and criticize their actions. Jesus reminds us to get the plank out of our own eye before showing our brother or sister the speck in his/her eye.

Matthew 7:1-5 (NLT) 7 "Do not judge others, and you will not be judged. 2 For you will be treated as you treat others.[a] The standard you use in judging is the standard by which you will be judged.[b] 3 "And why worry about a speck in your friend's eye[c] when you have a log in your own? 4 How can you think of saying to your friend,[d] 'Let me help you get rid of that speck in your eye,' when you can't see past the log in your own eye? 5 Hypocrite! First get rid of the log in your own eye; then you will see well enough to deal with the speck in your friend's eye."

You may need to constantly remind yourself that we have all sinned and fallen short of the glory of God. You may see a shortcoming in my life that God has not yet convicted me to deal with as of yet. This may be something you have already overcome and now feel entitled to judge me because I haven't *arrived* in that area. We all grow with God at different rates in an intimate, individual walk with Him. You can be sure that some of the shortcomings you observe in others are still there most likely because God is currently working with that person on something more pivotal for his/her walk with Jesus. Even if God is speaking to that person about that particular part of their old nature, it is not our job to decide when and how they will have victory and grow in the faith. Meditate on this...If you can see an irritating behavior in someone else, could it be that God is trying to also work that same behavior out of you?

Breaking agreement with self-righteousness was big for me personally. Feelings of judgement were directly connected to my desire to eat after dinner. If this is an area in which you struggle, press in with the Lord about Proverbs 18:20-21. I chose the English standard version of the bible for this verse because it is quite clear in it's meaning:

Proverbs 18:20-21 (ESV) 20" From the fruit of a man's mouth his stomach is satisfied; he is satisfied by the yield of his lips. 21 Death and life are in the power of the tongue, and those who love it will eat its fruits."

Is your stomach not satisfied because of what you are thinking and speaking all day? The more I walked in love and not judgement, the less I possessed an empty feeling in my stomach. These cravings come from all the unhealthy thoughts you have going on in your head all day regarding others. Have you been mulling over what you expect from your spouse or children, coworkers or friends in your head all day long? Have you had conversations in your head with these people and these conversations never took place? Most of these rehearsed scenarios and conversations are birthed out of expectations you have of others. This is another form of fretting.

Fretting falls under the category of *stinkin' thinkin'*. All of these unhealthy thoughts are not going to produce good things coming out of your mouth. Luke reminds us how our thoughts are attached to our heart:

Luke 6:45 (NLT) "A good person produces good things from the treasury of a good heart, and an evil person produces evil things from the treasury of an evil heart. What you say flows from what is in your heart."

How can you begin to deal with this sin? Confess your thoughts of judgement toward others as you catch them. Ask the Holy Spirit to give you an inward witness when your mind goes into fretting or worrying over what others are doing (or not doing). When the Holy Spirit brings fretting and judgement to your attention, you can quickly confess and change the thought to something praiseworthy. Remind yourself of this very often quoted verse:

Philippians 4:8-9 (NLT) 8 "And now, dear brothers and sisters, one final thing. Fix your thoughts on what is true, and honorable, and right, and pure, and lovely, and admirable. Think about things that are excellent and worthy of praise. 9 Keep putting into practice all you learned and received from me-everything you heard from me and saw me doing. Then the God of peace will be with you."

The promise in Philippians 4:9 says that if you practice what verse 8 commands, *then the God of peace will be with you.* You can't have judgement and peace at the same time. Let's move on to the next weight producing emotion which is:

3. Anger - the definition is: *having extreme displeasure toward others or yourself.*

If you are dealing with anger, hatred, rage, etc, This can cause you to gain weight as a defense mechanism to keep others away. When you are dealing with anger, it is hard to not dwell on the situation or person that is causing the anger. Those thoughts will drive you to feel bad about yourself and you'll want to drown the feelings. If you tend to overeat, you most likely will pacify yourself with food. The Apostle, Paul wrote to the believers in Colossae regarding anger and other unhealthy responses:

Colossians 3:8-10 (NLT) 8 "But now is the time to get rid of anger, rage, malicious behavior, slander and dirty language. 9 Don't lie to each other, for you have stripped off your old sinful nature and all its wicked deeds. 10 Put on your new nature, and be renewed as you learn to know your Creator and become like Him."

Food diverts you from feeling the emotion, to focusing on the food. The food is meant to silence the feelings and it temporarily does for some people. Someone once said, "when you bury feelings, you bury them alive." You can guarantee that anger and resentment you just swallowed with your ice cream is alive and well. Those feelings are like taking a live hand grenade and pulling the pin out. You will have no control over when and where that bomb will explode. You may choose to not deal with those emotions today, but eventually you will need to if you want to have a healthy body and soul. Anger can often lead you to the next unhealthy emotion, which is guilt.

4. Guilt - The definition is *a bad feeling caused by knowing or thinking that you have done something bad or wrong.* Guilt often accompanies emotional overeating. You may be experiencing guilt because you have an inward witness (from your conscience) that the anger you are holding is not from God. The guilt often causes you to overeat. You may hear an accusing voice with every bite saying something like, "You will be sorry you ate this when you get on the scale tomorrow." This adds yet another layer of guilt and self-condemnation and will keep you in a viscous cycle. The guilt and condemnation just drive you back to eating again for comfort.

One of the keys to stopping this sort of emotional eating cycle is if you begin to feel self-pity, self-righteousness and/or anger and sense that you are about to medicate with food, stop and give yourself permission to feel the emotions that you are so desperately running away from. Allow those negative responses to wash over you briefly. Reason them out with the Lord.

Ephesians 4 tells us when we are angry, to not sin.

Ephesians 4:26 (TLB) " *If you are angry, don't sin by nursing your grudge. Don't let the sun go down with you still angry—get over it quickly."*

It's okay to be angry or have a moment of self-pity. It's what your next step is that determines whether you will self-medicate with food. God gave us emotions. They are tools for our use, not to be shoved behind a door or choked down with a bag of chips. Most people no longer feel the need to eat when they have allowed themselves to work through their discontent and concern with the Lord.

What other areas can cause discontent in your life? How about gossip? My favorite definition of gossip is, *When two or more people stand in agreement with the lies of the enemy.* As a Christian, there is no way you feel good about yourself after you have just gossiped. Gossip is a major guilt trigger and rightfully so. Your own conscience condemns you. Proverbs has much to say about the subjects of the conscience and it gives many wise words about gossip. Let's examine a few of these wise sayings:

Proverbs 20:27 says, *(NLT) "The Lord's light penetrates the human spirit exposing every hidden motive."*

Proverbs 18:20 says, *(NLT) "Wise words satisfy like a good meal; the right words bring satisfaction."*

Proverbs 12:18 says,*(NLT) " Some people make cutting remarks, but the words of the wise bring healing."*

There are quite a few proverbs that indicate that our stomach is satisfied by the fruit of our mouth (or what we speak). Do you experience cravings when you really aren't hungry? Could it be that you were speaking unholy things about another person that day? Is your stomach not satisfied because your lips produced something that left you empty? Is there guilt in your heart because your conscience convicted you?

What comes out of your mouth determines, to a degree, what goes in it. If you are an emotional eater, what you are speaking will determine what and how much you are eating.

How about your thoughts of others? Maybe you are careful not to gossip but have many conversations in your head with people you are angry, bitter toward or annoyed with because of something they have said or not said. Those conversations are a form of fretting. I touched on fretting briefly under self-righteousness but this is what Psalm 37 says about the subject:

Psalm 37:1-6 (NLT) 1 "Don't worry (fret) about the wicked or envy those who do wrong. 2 For like grass, they soon fade away. 3 Trust in the Lord and do good. Then you will live safely in the land and prosper. 4 Take delight in the Lord, and He will give you your heart's desires. 5 Commit everything you do to the Lord. Trust Him and He will help you. 6 He will make your innocence radiate like the dawn, and the justice of your cause will shine like the noonday sun."

The problem with these conversations is that they haven't even happened yet and most of those conversations never will happen, but they cause all kinds of torment and upsetment in your spirit. If you are experiencing any of these conversations currently in your head, it is vital that you take it all before your Maker and reason it out with Him. He will be faithful to show you any unholy expectations you are carrying toward the person (or people) who have offended you. What is so dangerous about fretting is that your subconscious cannot tell the difference between reality and what is just happening in your thoughts. The subconscious mind stores all of your life experiences, your beliefs, your memories, your skills, all situations you've been through and all images you've ever seen. As you fret, you are storing situations that never even happened in your subconscious. Your mind actually thinks these situations and conversations are reality! This is very damaging to those relationships with the people you are fretting about. Social media can be a stumbling block for fretting. I personally had to disconnect from Facebook for two and a half years until I could learn to not absorb what I witnessed other people post. I must admit that every once in a while, someone can still disturb my peace in this arena.

As you are pressing in with God about your fretting, ask yourself some questions: "Did I let the sun go down on my anger?" "Did I let a root of bitterness spring up?" "Am I judging a person or people for what they are (or aren't) doing?" "Am I fretting over a Facebook or Twitter post?" If the answer to any of the above is "yes," it is your responsibility before the Lord to ask for forgiveness for allowing the enemy's tools to be used against you.

Colossians 3:8-9 (ESV) covers a lot of what is in satan's tool box: *8 "But now you must put them all away: anger, wrath, malice, slander, and obscene talk from your mouth. 9 Do not lie to one another, seeing that you have put off the old self[a] with its practices."*

Then Colossians 3:10-14 gives us the antidote for our issues with others;

Colossians 3:10-14 (NLT) 10 "Put on your new nature, and be renewed as you learn to know your Creator and become like him. 11 In this new life, it doesn't matter if you are a Jew or a Gentile,[a] circumcised or uncircumcised, barbaric, uncivilized,[b] slave, or free. Christ is all that matters, and he lives in all of us. 12 Since God chose you to be the holy people he loves, you must clothe yourselves with tenderhearted mercy, kindness, humility, gentleness, and patience. 13 Make allowance for each other's faults, and forgive anyone who offends you. Remember, the Lord forgave you, so you must forgive others. 14 Above all, clothe yourselves with love, which binds us all together in perfect harmony."

If the peace of God is ruling in your heart, you won't need the oral fix (emotional comfort food) to quiet the voices in your head.

5. Loneliness - This emotion can also be a key factor in comfort eating. Loneliness is not a sin. It is not wrong to want to have a spouse, more friends, family who wants to spend time with you, etc. Ask yourself, "What am I doing with the time when the feelings of loneliness hit?" Are you reaching out? Are you one who puts expectations on others to do the calling and reaching out to you? As a believer, are you filling that empty space (that only God can fill) with prayer, Bible reading and/or worship and praise. The Word says that the Lord inhabits the praise of His people. If you are praising God, then you are not alone. God is with you in the room. There is no earthly company that can compare to Jesus.

John 14:16 (NLT) says, "And I will ask the Father, and He will give you another Advocate, who will never leave you."

The Holy Spirit is with you all of the time living inside of you; if you have accepted Jesus Christ as your Lord and Savior.

I am in no way trying to diminish your need for human contact. God made us to be interdependent on others and to be relational. We are not to be alone all of the time. Could there be some key reasons why you are experiencing loneliness? Conduct an honest evaluation of yourself. Are you easy to be around? Do you lift others up? Do you talk about what is aggravating you instead of focusing on the positive aspects of life?

Philippians 4:8(NLT) "And now, dear brothers and sisters, one final thing. Fix your thoughts on what is true, and honorable and right, and pure, and lovely and admirable. Think about things that are excellent and worthy of praise."

It is draining to be around others who only share the drama and strife that is happening in their lives. The more you talk about your drama, the more you stir up trouble in your mind and in your atmosphere. Do you want to be known as the person who sucks the life out of others? Are you the person who talks so much that no one else can get a word in? When a friend shares a story or experience, do you have to compare your own or are you content to just listen? If you are feeling the Holy Spirit conviction, go before the Lord and ask for forgiveness for being exhausting to be around. Ask Him to renew your mind as you delve into His Word for healing. Study the gospels. I would encourage you to take an in-depth look at how Jesus interacted with other human beings.

6. Martyr - How about emotional eating due to playing the role of Martyr? Martyrs of this type are those who exaggerate their difficulties in order to obtain

sympathy from others. Can you identify with him/her? This person who holds everything in? Everyone in your home becomes an emotional hostage as you cast silent judgement on them. Your silence (and sometimes not so silent dish slamming, or huffing, or sighing under your breath) makes everyone wary of you. You may sense when everyone is *walking on eggshells* around you and you take pleasure in it. You have rationalized in your mind that you are the one who does the lion's share of the work in your home, work place, church group or PTA. You have allowed bitterness, resentment, and maybe even unforgiveness to creep in.

What does all of this have to do with overeating? If you can identify with the traits of martyrdom, it witnesses to your spirit that you emotionally eat as a result of this self-imposed prison. I say self-imposed because you have chosen this position of bondage even though you are a free person in Christ. You may be saying to yourself right now; "But nobody helps me, nobody cares, nobody sees how much is on my shoulders." God knows and He sees. Ask Him for ways to express your discouragement with others in a gentle, loving way; then thank *Him* for changing the hearts of those around you. It is difficult to want to help someone who is always angry. Most people just want to run and hide. Decide right now that you no longer want to be a martyr in your home, church group, work environment, or anywhere else for that matter. Ask for forgiveness from the Lord for your behavior. You may need to humble yourself and ask the people you have held in bondage with your attitude to forgive you as well. Ask for the wisdom to display healthy emotion in these areas where you have played the martyr/victim. You may also want to take a look at your schedule and see if there are events, programs, activities that God never asked you to do in the first place. Repent and get out from under those areas as soon as possible. You will begin to get comfortable with the Lord and realize that you don't need to fill every minute of your time to feel like a worthwhile human being. Resting in the Lord is pivotal to staying out of the martyr/victim role.

7. Jealousy and covetousness: These two emotions basically mean, *feeling resentment because of another's success or advantages*. Do these reactions cause a person to overeat? Absolutely. God's word says to "Seek ye first the Kingdom of God and all these things shall be added unto you." What that means is, if God is in His rightful place as King of your life, He will give you the desires of your heart. When you give Him your first fruits, seeking the infilling with Bible, prayer, and worship, your fleshly desires will begin to fall and He will have room in your heart to implant His desires for your life. Your selfish wants will naturally fade away. His ways are higher than yours. Don't you want to replace your fleshly desires for what God wants to give you? He will give you a peace and a purpose like you have never had before! Then when new desires rise up in your heart, you will know that they are of Him and you can be assured that they will come to pass.

Ecclesiastes 5:10-11 (NLT) says, 10 "Those who love money will never have enough. How meaningless to think that wealth brings true happiness! 11 The more you have, the more people will come to spend it. So what good is wealth - except perhaps to watch it slip through your fingers?"

There is a deception in the prosperity message that says, "The King's kids should have the best of everything." I am all for God's favor and proclaim it out loud, but there is a fine line between the favor and prosperity of God and thinking that you are entitled to the best of everything all of the time in every circumstance. This forsakes wise counsel regarding finances. Paul said, "I have learned to be content in much and in little." We must learn the same. Let any seeds of desire be planted by the Lord and not by your wondering eye and jealousy of what others have. It will give you one less reason to self-medicate with food.

Can you see how your thoughts and the words you speak affect your eating?

At one point during my personal journey with food bondage, I felt the urging of the Holy Spirit to look up the definition of *oral fixation*. It means *the obsessive interest relating to the mouth*. I was seeking to pacify the feelings connected to a problem or argument by grabbing a bag of chips or a pint of ice cream. Commercials on television teach us to do this. How many times have you seen a movie or TV show where the "just jilted" woman/man is comforting herself/himself with a pint of ice cream? This is a big area of concern for most people, so I am urging you to linger over the prayer below and really press in with the Lord about your emotions. I believe there are huge keys in being set free from the bondage of emotional eating here. I urge you not to lightly skip over this prayer or say it in a rote fashion. Doing so will not produce the results that the Lord has waiting just for you! This is where I love to see God's people have a sense of entitlement! We are seated with Christ in heavenly places. Believe that in prayer you are entitled to destroy the power that these unhealthy emotions have had over your life and your weight!

Prayer: Dear Lord, I come to You convicted of how I have allowed my emotions to run my thought life. I ask You by the power of Your Holy Spirit to show me every area that I need to confess as an area of sin (e.g.; self-pity, judgement, resentment, anger, loneliness, jealousy, etc). If there are open doors from my past, I ask you to illuminate them. (Wait for the Holy Spirit to show you any open doors from your past.) I desire every door that is currently open to the enemy to be shut so I will gain victory over my emotional eating patterns. Wash me in Your love. In Jesus' name I pray, Amen.

As the Lord shows you each area, ask Him for forgiveness. Then confess out loud, "Lord, I break agreement with (whatever areas He has shown you) in Jesus' name."

Psalms 32:1-11 (NLT)

Psalm 32A psalm[a] of David.

1 "Oh, what joy for those whose disobedience is forgiven, whose sin is put out of sight! 2 Yes, what joy for those whose record the Lord has cleared of guilt,[b] whose lives are lived in complete honesty! 3 When I refused to confess my sin, my body wasted away, and I groaned all day long. 4 Day and night Your hand of discipline was heavy on me. My strength evaporated like water in the summer heat. Interlude 5 Finally, I confessed all my sins to You and stopped trying to hide my guilt. I said to myself, "I will confess my rebellion to the Lord." And You forgave me! All my guilt is gone. Interlude 6 Therefore, let all the godly pray to You while there is still time, that they may not drown in the floodwaters of judgment. 7 For You are my hiding place; You protect me from trouble. You surround me with songs of victory. Interlude 8 The Lord says, "I will guide you along the best pathway for your life. I will advise you and watch over you. 9 Do not be like a senseless horse or mule that needs a bit and bridle to keep it under control." 10 Many sorrows come to the wicked, but unfailing love surrounds those who trust the Lord. 11 So rejoice in the Lord and be glad, all you who obey Him! Shout for joy, all you whose hearts are pure!"

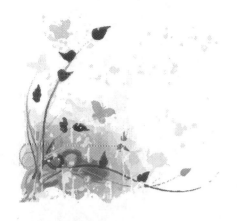

Notes

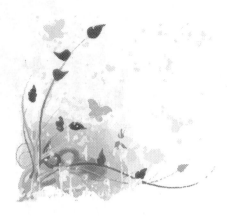

Inner Vows

If you looked at the title of this chapter and asked the question, "What in the world is an inner vow?" you are not alone. If you are not familiar with this terminology, inner vows are the statements you made to yourself about what you would or would not ever allow in your own life. It basically means that you observe a behavior in another person and judge it as not okay in your own life. Based on that decision, then you determine that it will NEVER happen for you. For example, as a child you may have had parents that would not ever allow candy/sugar in your home. You may have vowed to yourself that when you have kids, you will allow them to have candy, cookies, etc. whenever they want! An inner vow is set in the mind and the heart. Inner vows resist change and can stunt your maturity. You don't grow out of the inner vows made as a child or teenager. They hold so much power because we don't usually remember or recognize them as vows. As a result, they become finely woven into our character.

This chapter is dedicated to rooting out those inner vows that may be holding you back from giving the Lord your appetite for food. You will also discover any vows that keep you chained to the desires to conform to the world. As you work through this chapter, you will find many questions that you need to ask yourself. I encourage you to write down your answers for your prayer time at the end of this chapter in the section provided.

Many of these vows are made as children or teenagers and are deeply rooted. Let's explore some more examples of inner vows. Many young girls and boys who have been molested or raped, will often make inner vows. After such a traumatic event (or series of events), these children may vow to NEVER allow another person to have control over them again. They may state such an oath out loud or it may just be a thought that results in a decision in their minds. Now, let's take a look at how that oath may affect their lives as adults. These people may have much difficulty in submitting to any authority put over them (even a boss in the workplace). A serious root of rebellion can be the result of the oath/vow made many years ago. Let's look at another example. Maybe you have had a spouse who committed adultery. Maybe you have forgiven him/her but vowed never to allow that person (or anyone else) to ever get that close to you again. The vow seemed like the only logical way to protect yourself. You never wanted to experience a repeat of such pain of betrayal ever again. Or suppose you lived in a family where your parents yelled at each other often. You may have vowed not to be in a verbally abusive or loud relationship. Sounds good, right? The flaw in this vow is that you may run from conflict instead of handling it in a healthy manner.

These vows may seem good or useful at the time they are made. They do, however, come back to haunt you as an adult. Sometimes you are judging others and making the vow out of a sense of self-righteousness. Jesus forbids oaths (vows) in the book of Matthew.

Matthew 5:33-37 (NLT) 33 "You have also heard that our ancestors were told, 'You must not break your vows; you must carry out the vows you make to the Lord.'[a] 34 But I say, do not make any vows! Do not say, 'By heaven!' because heaven is God's throne. 35 And do not say, 'By the earth!' because the earth is His footstool. And do not say, 'By Jerusalem!' for Jerusalem is the city of the great King. 36 Do not even say, 'By my head!' for you can't turn one hair white or black. 37 Just say a simple, 'Yes, I will,' or 'No, I won't.' Anything beyond this is from the evil one."

The definition of a vow or an oath is *a solemn promise about one's future actions or behavior.* It is a sworn declaration. When you make vows, you are basically saying, "I am the only one who can be trusted. I am the only one who can take care of me and upon whom I can rely." You begin to push other people and most importantly, God, out of the picture. If you are compelled to make a vow, you don't trust God in that area of your life. These types of inner vows are *self-preservation* vows. A declaration like this also gives the enemy an open door due to your rebellion. If you are a victim of rape or molestation and do not seek help, you will most likely erect walls around yourself and never let anyone fully in once the inner vow has been established. What happens if or when such unhealed people marry? The marriage covenant can only be partly fulfilled, thereby leaving an area for the other partner to hit that wall of self-protection and feel neglected as a result.

In the instance where there was a vow made in a verbally abusive home, the person may avoid confrontation and even avoid healthy discussions at all costs out of a fear and determination that there will be no yelling in **their** home. This can open doors to roots of bitterness and unforgiveness. No human being on this earth can swallow that much unresolved conflict without ramifications. You can be sure that in a home like this the sun has gone down on anger plenty of times. How should anger be handled? Ephesians gives you some insight:

Ephesians 4:25-27 (NLT) 25 "So stop telling lies. Let us tell our neighbors the truth, for we are all parts of the same body. 26 And "don't sin by letting anger control you."[a] don't let the sun go down while you are still angry, 27 for anger gives a foothold to the devil."

Can you see how an inner vow can hurt you? As a Christian you are to be moving toward a place of total surrender to the Lord. Each of us will move toward that goal in God's timing by the unction of the Holy Spirit. As the Lord shows you these areas, you need to surrender them. You have a choice. God gave you free will. Will you comply with His gentle leading? Sometimes you want to, but you can't seem to fight your flesh (the spirit is willing but the flesh is weak.) Difficulty obeying the Lord can be a result of one or more inner vows you made so long ago that you don't even realize the vows are there. The vows became a part of who you are and how you operate with others and with God. It can be an unspoken vow or a trapped thought that, until now, you weren't cognitively aware of. A trapped thought is a statement that is usually untrue and plays over and over in your mind. You may not even be aware of how often these thoughts come into your mind on a daily basis. Take a moment to write down any thoughts that the Holy Spirit is bringing to your attention.

How do inner vows cause food issues? Some cravings for food are rooted in inner vows. What exactly are cravings? The Oxford English Dictionary describes them as, *a powerful desire for something.* The picture on the next page was drawn by a talented young artist who depicted Eve as half woman and half pig.

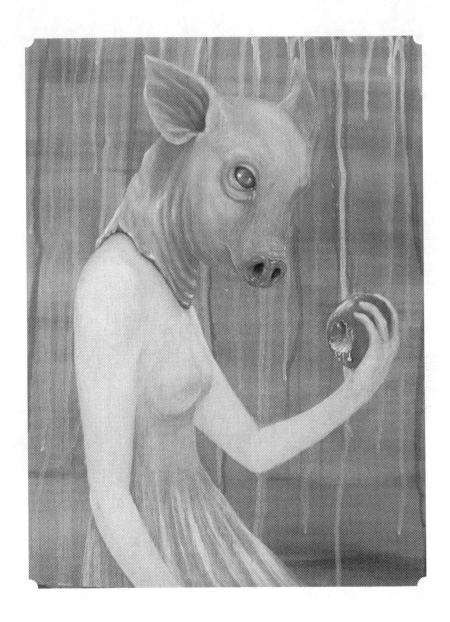

It is a shocking picture, but if you think about Eve's craving (powerful desire) for knowledge from the tree of the knowledge of good and evil, it inspired this young artist to draw her as insatiable.

Did the enemy whisper into Eve's ear that she didn't need God (or Adam for that matter)? Did he tell her what she should and shouldn't eat that day? She bought into his lies. Could this be why women seem to struggle with food issues more than men? I personally believe the struggle started for us in the garden.

What lies has the enemy whispered into your ear? Do any of these sound familiar?

1. I won't be truly beautiful until I am thin.
2. When I am at my goal weight, then I will be happy.
3. No one will ever want me if I am fat.
4. I am not worth anything with these extra pounds on me.
5. No one will ever be able to love me this way.
6. I am weak and have no power over sweets or cravings.
7. I will be good at sports when I am thin.
8. People don't want to be around me or be seen with me because I am fat.

These trapped thoughts can lead to inner vows like:

1. Maybe you stood in judgement of someone else and vowed, "I will never be fat and disgusting like my Mom, Dad, friend, etc."
2. Maybe you were the thin kid who bullied the fat kids and vowed to never look like them or to ever be a victim like them.

3. Maybe you were that bullied, chubby kid who vowed that you were determined to get the weight off no matter what it took, even if you had to punish your body to do it. Maybe it lead to an eating disorder to fulfill your inner vow to yourself.

4. Maybe you were the molested or raped child mentioned earlier and have erected a wall of weight around yourself in an effort to keep people at arm's length.

You make an inner vow from a place of hurt, anger, judgement and even a need for revenge. Maybe your inner vow was an open door to an eating disorder. Maybe throwing up or starving yourself was the only way to keep your vow and prove to yourself and others you could be what they said you could *never* be. You need to ask forgiveness for making these inner vows.

Consider your own life as you read the testimony of my dear friend:

As a child I lived in constant fear. My father's moods would shift like the wind. We walked on eggshells, always afraid that a word or glance would send him into a rage. I was always the target. The feeling of fear began to manifest itself in many ways. I was not allowed to show emotion. I didn't dare cry or make a sound; so I swallowed it. Then fear settled into my belly. I had learned to pretend that he didn't scare me and I was able to look unafraid, but my stomach would be in a constant state of gnawing. I had a sick feeling of emptiness so I began to eat. The food was like a soothing balm. I shook from fear as I ate and once it hit my belly and filled the empty, gnawing space, it calmed me down.

I soon realized that my father controlled everything in my life including my emotions. One thing he could not control was what I ate and my weight. My father hated and was disgusted by anyone who was fat. If they were rotund, he told them so. I became the one thing he hated the most, *fat*. I felt powerful like I was getting him back for all that he had done to me. But really I was only hurting myself. The bondage to food, coupled with my inner vow, would continue for forty five years. I would feel powerful in one way but experience self-hate simultaneously. I was caught between two emotions and neither one of them was healthy.

Recently after doing a Bible study on weight loss with a focus on getting to the root of the problem, I realized that when I would get the gnawing feeling in my stomach it was fear! It was the fear that I had felt constantly as a child. I felt like a light bulb had gone on in my mind after all of these years.

I spent my whole life eating to quench the gnawing feeling in my belly. Maybe sometimes it was real hunger, but it would remind me of that helpless feeling I felt as a child. The goal was always to make the emptiness disappear quickly. As I slowly began to speak to my soul and physical body that it was okay to feel hungry, I reminded myself that I wasn't starving and there was also no reason to fear. I would tell myself that I was no longer a small child living with an angry man. I cannot begin to express the life changing healing that began to take place. I thought back to my childhood. I could not control what was taking place. I was small. I had a father that raged and was so wounded himself that he hurt others. With this revelation, as an adult I can now control how I feel. I know that fear does not run my life and that it is not from God. The Lord is my protector and my healer. No longer will I be afraid.

1 John 1:9 says (NLT) "But if we confess our sins to him, he is faithful and just to forgive us our sins and to cleanse us from all wickedness.

My dear friend's story exposes a conglomeration of trapped thoughts and inner vows. One trapped thought was thinking the food would soothe her belly. She now knows that the Lord is her comforter and not food. Her inner vow was she determined to get her dad back by being what he hated most - fat. The Lord was faithful to show her the roots of her eating problem and she is experiencing freedom today.

Sit quietly before the Lord and pray this prayer and ask for His divine revelation to expose and break the trapped thoughts and inner vows.

Dear Heavenly Father, I thank You for revealing all truth to me. I come to You now as Your child knowing that no good thing will You withhold from me according to Psalm 84:11. Your word says, "If any of us lacks wisdom, we are to ask and You will freely give it." (James 1:5). I am asking, as I pray, that You expose and pull up any hidden inner vows I made. Please illuminate any trapped thoughts I have that allow the enemy to have territory in this area of my life. I ask this in Jesus' name.

If you have your heavenly prayer language, please pray in the Spirit. This bypasses your earthly mind and thoughts and allows the Holy Spirit to gently pull up situations or circumstances that led to establishing the inner vows. If you do not have tongues, sit quietly and trust the Lord to speak to you.

Ask the Lord to forgive you for making the vow(s) out of ignorance, rebellion, anger, etc. Then break agreement with the vow(s) one by one saying out loud; "I break agreement with the inner vow I made that stated _____(you fill in the blank) (e.g.," I will never let anyone control me again" or "I will be thin no matter what it takes.") I apply the Blood of Jesus to that vow. Forgive me for relying on myself and not on You, Lord. I believe I am set free by the Blood of the Lamb. In Jesus' name, amen."

Wait on God until you believe everything He wants you to pray over and break agreement with is taken care of. You may experience a sense of release or a feeling of just being lighter. If you do not feel anything after your prayer time, please do not feel defeated. If you broke the vows and trapped thoughts with your mouth and asked for forgiveness, you are walking in a new freedom.

The other pivotal part of this prayer is applying the Blood of Jesus to the vow. I really want you to take hold of the knowledge that His Blood is of the *yoke-bearing, burden destroying* kind! His blood is still warm, it's still alive, it still saves, heals and delivers. When you utilize His precious Blood by applying it to an old bondage, it sets you free. Begin to thank and praise Him even now for His life-giving blood that never runs out!

As a Spirit-filled believer, you may be accustomed to relying on your feelings or emotions to dictate whether the Spirit is working in your life. You need to believe that the prayer of a righteous man (and woman) can accomplish much just like the Word says in James 5:16. You are not to base your walk with the most high God on just feelings and emotions. Believe that you are now walking in the resurrection power (that same power that rose Christ from the dead) in those areas that you just broke agreement with.

This belief will propel you forward to the next chapter about worry and how it effects your relationship with food.

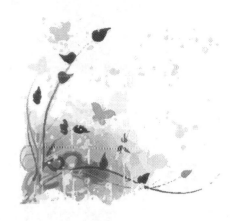

Notes

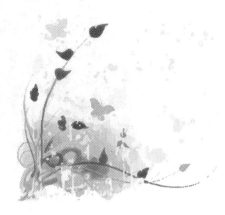

Chapter 4

Do Not Worry

Matthew 6:25 (NLT) "This is why I tell you not to worry about everyday life - whether you have enough food and drink, or enough clothes to wear. Isn't life more than food, and your body more than clothing?"

In case you haven't noticed by now, I love to research the actual meaning of words in the dictionary. You will find that each chapter contains definitions of various words. Their meanings are important. The definition of worry is *to feel or cause to feel troubled over actual or possible difficulties.*

Do you worry about food? Do you wake up every day determined to have your eating under control? Do you determine that you will eat only certain food groups that day? Do you jump on every new diet that makes headlines? Do you have very strong opinions about not allowing certain foods to pass through your lips? Do you visualize some foods as being extremely harmful to your body? Do you cast judgmental eyes on someone as they are scarfing down a cheeseburger and fries, or a non-organic fruit or a sugar laden candy bar?

I confess that at one time or another throughout my life I have walked in all of these worries! Romans Chapter 8 declares our freedom:

Romans 8: 9-17 (NLT) 9 "But you are not controlled by your sinful nature. You are controlled by the Spirit if you have the Spirit of God living in you. (And remember that those who do not have the Spirit of Christ living in them do not belong to Him at all.) 10 And Christ lives within you, so even though your body will die because of sin, the Spirit gives you life[a] because you have been made right with God. 11 The Spirit of God, who raised Jesus from the dead, lives in you. And just as God raised Christ Jesus from the dead, he will give life to your mortal bodies by this same Spirit living within you.

12 Therefore, dear brothers and sisters,[b] you have no obligation to do what your sinful nature urges you to do. 13 For if you live by its dictates, you will die. But if through the power of the Spirit you put to death the deeds of your sinful nature,[c] you will live. 14 For all who are led by the Spirit of God are children[d] of God. 15 So you have not received a spirit that makes you fearful slaves. Instead, you received God's Spirit when He adopted you as His own children.[e] Now we call Him, "Abba, Father."[f] 16 For His Spirit joins with our spirit to affirm that we are God's children. 17 And since we are His children, we are His heirs. In fact, together with Christ we are heirs of God's glory. But if we are to share His glory, we must also share His suffering."

You are to walk in the Spirit and not in the flesh. Even as a believer I know I was definitely walking in the flesh. My thoughts were consumed with what to eat, when to eat it, why I was eating it and how I was eating it. I constantly worried about and monitored my weight.

While in counselor training classes, I chose to do a book report on Lisa Bevere's book, *You Are Not What You Weigh*. It was just what I needed. I realized that I had made food an idol. The scale determined how much self-esteem I had for the day and I had come into agreement with food bondage. My food bondage dictated that if it wasn't organic, it was harmful. If it contained sodium nitrates, it would promote cancer. If it had too much sugar, it would wear down my immune system. The list goes on and on. My thoughts were consumed. I was worshipping at the altar of self-preservation. As I read the chapters, I repented for the idols I had erected and asked the Lord to heal my thinking. I fasted a few days and gave what I would have eaten to a family who needed it. Isaiah gives us insight as to why you should share your food with the needy when fasting:

Isaiah 58:10 (NLT) "Feed the hungry, and help those in trouble. Then your light will shine out from the darkness, and the darkness around you will be as bright as noon."

During that time I meditated on Isaiah 58 and what the Lord says about fasting. When the fast was over I began to live Isaiah 58:11:

Isaiah 58:11 (NLT) "The Lord will guide you continually, giving you water when you are dry and restoring your strength. You will be like a well-watered garden, like an ever-flowing spring."

I allowed the Lord to guide my eating. I asked Him to tell me what to eat as I went about my day. If I was not hearing from Him clearly, I would ask Him to help me have a desire for what He wanted me to eat. I walked in a new freedom! My relationship to food changed. I found that my body needed much less than I had been eating. I was satisfied. I would take long breaks from the scale. The scale would no longer rule how I felt about myself on a daily basis.

I did meal planning for my family as I always had done but now was eating much less and feeling satisfied. One of the new behaviors I adopted helped me to break out of old patterns of needing something sweet right after dinner. I would immediately make myself a cup of hot, fruit flavored tea. I drink mine without sweetener, but putting a little honey or the sweetener of your choice in your tea would definitely be less sugar and fewer calories than having a dessert. The warm tea brought comfort and completion to my meal while I was still in the process of breaking off the old pattern.

I had torn down my idols but was still battling some old patterns. You may find that you will have to walk out certain areas of your healing as well. I had been eating dessert after dinner my entire life. My mom was a great cook and my dad loved her desserts. She made wonderful cakes, pies, cookies, etc. Dessert was always available in our home and had become a source of comfort in my life. As I drank the tea, it would help me remember that I no longer needed sweets as a symbol of love or completion to a meal. The tendency to need dessert has been long gone and it is a wonderful place of freedom to experience!

I would love to tell you about my friend. Her name is Rachel. She is a lovely, young lady in her twenties and she battled greatly with eating issues. Here is her testimony:

I had struggled most of my life with anorexia, binge eating, purging, over-exercising, and yo yo dieting. I didn't know how to eat right. What was a normal portion size? How can I eat in moderation? How can I stop eating when I

am no longer hungry? How do I know what to buy at the grocery store? Donna, my counselor and friend, shared an eating concept with me "Pray and ask the Holy Spirit to show you what to eat," she explained. "But how do I know if it is the Holy Spirit or if it is me?" I asked. Donna explained it to me in detail; so I began this eating concept. I prayed first thing in the morning. As I prayed, I asked the Holy Spirit to show me what to eat for breakfast, how much to eat, and when to eat it. It worked the very first day I tried it! I would get a healthy desire (not an obsessive desire) to eat something. God would either highlight it in the refrigerator, or tell me in my spirit what to eat. After dinner is usually the most difficult time for me because I crave carbs and sugar before bed. The first day I tried this spiritual eating concept, right before bed when the cravings came, I called on The Holy Spirit for help. I ask Him what I should do. Should I eat anything at all I wondered? The Holy Spirit reminded me of the banana chips I had forgotten about in the cabinet. "Just a handful," I felt God say. So I portioned out just a handful. I had a craving for tea suddenly and made a warm cup of decaf chai tea. As I sat on the couch relaxing with my tea and small handful of banana chips, I felt completely at peace with no guilt. When I was finished, I felt totally satisfied with no more cravings.

I experienced and still do experience days like this every time I use this eating concept that Donna shared with me. I have actually lost weight using this concept. It has been a slow process, but I feel so proud of myself and the weight is staying off. Have there been moments of weakness where I have not listened to the Holy Spirit? Yes there have been; however, I asked God to help me get back on track and it is always a peaceful experience. Before, if I got off track with my eating, I would always tear myself apart and be so hard and unforgiving of myself.

I'm so grateful that by utilizing this eating concept and other spiritual tools Donna has shared with me, I am finally on my journey to wholeness and healing and I feel a little bit more free everyday!

Rachel

Rachel is a success story and her story can be your success story too!

Some of you have already conquered this area with Christ, but have bought into a different lie. This lie says that everything you eat has to be healthy or it is harmful to your body. You may be basing this on *1 Corinthians 6:19-20 (NLT) 19 "Don't you realize that your body is the temple of the Holy Spirit, who lives in you and was given to you by God? You do not belong to yourself, 20 for God bought you with a high price. So you must honor God with your body."*

If you read the whole chapter, you will see that Paul was saying sexual immorality was more harmful than what we eat.

Are you to take good care of your body? Yes! You are however, not to fall into bondage because of it. You must find balance in this area of eating. You must be able to adjust to what is available to eat. Let's take some lessons from the Word.

1 Corinthians 10:-23-25 (NLT) 23 "You say, "I am allowed to do anything"

(a) - but not everything is good for you. You say, "I am allowed to do anything" - but not everything is beneficial. 24 Don't be concerned for your own good but for the good of others. 25 So you may eat any meat that is sold in the marketplace without raising questions of conscience."

You may have the freedom of picking and choosing what you want to eat and that is wonderful. We may not always have that freedom in the days ahead. If you have the wrong mentality about what is acceptable to eat, you will struggle greatly if that time comes while you are still on the earth. Even in America, we may face future food shortages or have questionable things to eat. The Lord drove this point home with me by showing me that regardless if I am about to eat an organic apple or a donut, I am to thank Him and ask Him to bless it to my body in Jesus' name. He has shown me that I should visualize food blessing (healing, nourishing, etc) my entire body because of the prayer of faith and gratitude for the food He has given me.

This is not a license to choose unhealthy things to eat all the time and expect God to bail you out. You need the freedom of balance and freedom to not panic based on availability.

Let's take a look at some other scriptures that back up this line of thinking:

John 6:27 (NLT) "But don't be so concerned about perishable things like food. Spend your energy seeking the eternal life that the Son of Man can give you. For God the Father has given me the seal of His approval."

Mark 7:18-19 (NLT) 18 "Don't you understand either?" He asked. "Can't you see that the food you put into your body cannot defile you? 19 Food doesn't go into your heart, but only passes through the stomach and then goes into the sewer." (By saying this He declared that every kind of food is acceptable in God's eyes.)

Do these scriptures give you a license to eat junk food all day every day? God forbid. Food is given for enjoyment, nourishment and celebration. You need to balance out your thinking about food. You are probably out of balance if you refer to eating something as bad for you or good for you. Don't label foods as the enemy or the hero. Just follow the leading of the Holy Spirit and walk in freedom.

The Holy spirit may tell some of you to fast something in particular. This is usually to get that food (sometimes sugar, etc.) back into a healthy balance. Fasting something you crave can break the yoke of bondage it has over your life. Then under the gentle leading of the Holy Spirit, you can introduce that food back into your life in moderation and balance.

There is such freedom in declaring all things have been made clean by the Blood of Jesus. Break agreement with the trapped thoughts and mind sets that the world has put on you regarding food.

If you suffer from food allergies, press in with the Lord in this area. Ask Him to show you any areas that need healing. There are many good Christian writers who touch on spiritual roots of physical ailments including food allergies. Researching a Christian book web site or book store will provide such reading material.

Just take it day by day, meal by meal with the Lord at your side guiding you through. He has every hair on your head numbered and He cares about helping you with your eating. He will help you meal plan for your family and He will help you not to waste food as well. You will walk in a new ease that you have not experienced before. Our God is a God of peace and order.

Let me share Danielle's story: She had gastric bypass. If you are not familiar with the term, it is the surgery that has been all the rage for weight loss over the past decade here in America and abroad. Danielle had done remarkably well having lost over 250 pounds! At that point she hit a wall with her diet and weight loss. Danielle had conquered many of her triggers for overeating but still had not been able to get past what seemed to be a plateau. She was stuck for quite a long period of time after her major weight loss. Her doctor wanted her to lose at least 70 pounds more and the weight was no longer coming off so easily. I suggested she try the method of eating what she felt God was telling her to eat at every meal. The idea was very appealing to her but she was apprehensive about starting that day. Why? She was leaving on a three day weekend trip where every meal would have to be eaten in a restaurant. I asked her to try this method anyway asking the Holy Spirit to really guide her as to what to eat at each meal. Danielle utilized this method even having dinner one evening at The Cheesecake Factory. She got the baked potato soup and a salad. It filled her up and kept her satisfied until morning. When Danielle returned home from her trip, she decided to brave the scale. Much to her delight, she had lost six pounds over the weekend! Her plateau was broken and she began to see how much she could trust the Lord even in this area of her life! Danielle had also struggled with regulating her fats, carbs and proteins for the doctor, and under divine direction, this was also no longer an issue.

What she could never achieve in her own strength was easily attained with God.

How can this method work with more serious eating disorders? As I mentioned in previous chapters, bulimia and anorexia cause a person to need to have total control over their food intake. This is due to feeling totally out of control in another or all areas of one's life. In this chapter our friend, Rachel, suffered from both anorexia and bulimia in her lifetime. One of her triggers for binging and purging was feeling overwhelmed with responsibilities as a wife, mother and massage therapist. As Rachel pressed in with the Lord and prayed through the prayers in the prior chapters, she found much freedom. Now, Rachel was ready to allow God to tell her what to eat meal by meal. This is the text I received from Rachel after the first two days of eating with the Holy Spirit in control:

"The first day I tried this eating concept something really cool happened! I ate what God told me and I was totally satisfied and felt full with no cravings. The next day was really good too. Then I got overwhelmed with all of the things I had to do. I got summoned to jury duty, was trying to pack our apartment to move, was working on income taxes and had a very heavy massage schedule to boot." Rachel had learned her trigger was feeling overwhelmed. If she had not recognized her pattern, she may have dived full steam into a bingeing and purging episode. She quickly recovered and allowed God to direct her eating in the midst of overwhelm. Just like Rachel, you can take Him as your partner everyday to guide you and lead you in all truth.

I want to wrap up this chapter by summarizing: With the Lord you can break the mind sets that cause you to worry and fret about what to eat. Fast under the leading of the Lord. Ask Him if He wants you to fast and, if so, what should you fast and how long? Then it will be easier to follow the day to day unction of the Holy Spirit as to what to eat.

Dear Lord, I thank you that I am yours and You say your sheep hear Your voice. Forgive me for being consumed with thoughts of food. Forgive me for judging others for what they eat (or don't eat). Forgive me for wasting food and not walking in Your divine peace. I turn this area of my life over to You, Holy Spirit, and ask You to guide me daily. In Jesus' name I pray. Amen

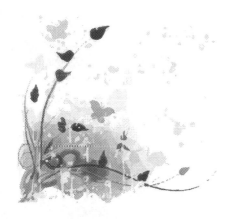

Notes

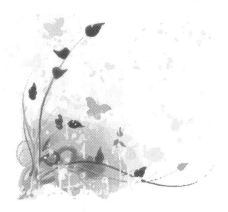

Chapter 5

Gluttony

The definition of gluttony is the habit or act of eating excessively. Unless you have lived in a third world country in serious poverty, I am guessing that you have overeaten to the point of feeling uncomfortable at least once in your life. Gluttony weighs a person down. It weighs down your spirit as well as your body.

Weight gain has mostly been the overlooked sin in the church. It seems to be more accepted than alcohol, drug abuse or homosexuality. Sin is sin in God's eyes and He is the judge. Do you view other addictions as more serious than a food addiction? For some of you, your weight has taken over your life just like an alcohol or drug problem. It has robbed you of your calling because you don't have the energy or aren't physically able to do what God has planned for you. Here is a thought on the subject from the writer of Proverbs 23:

Proverbs 23:20-21 (NLT) *"20 Do not carouse with drunkards or feast with gluttons, 21 for they are on their way to poverty, and too much sleep clothes them in rags."*

The Lord couples drunkenness with gluttony a few times in the Bible; so we have to assume that He considers one as offensive as the other. According to God's word, they lead to the same path. If this is speaking to you, take a moment to ask God to forgive you for judging the alcoholic, drug addict, adulterer, and murderer, etc. as a more serious sinner than you.

Take a personal inventory. Where do you personally stand with gluttony? Some of you overeat occasionally while others do it daily. Why? Perhaps you suffer from a fear of lack, fear of poverty or fear of loss of control. Perhaps you had an unstable environment growing up. Maybe you had times of no food in your house. Maybe as a young child you overheard your parent's conversations about not being able to pay the bills or buy groceries. Parents often speak poverty, lack, or fear of such things in ear-shot range of the children. As you hear these statements like "We can't afford that" and "Do you think money just grows on trees?" over and over again in your childhood, your little psyche can get hard-wired to focus on what you don't possess or can't afford instead of the wonderful things that **God is** supplying. These repetitive statements can be open doors for the enemy to plant fear of lack which can affect you as an adult. Let's take a look at what God spoke through the prophet Ezekiel regarding gluttony:

Ezekiel 16:49 (NLT) " Sodom's sins were pride, gluttony, and laziness, while the poor and needy suffered outside her door."

I don't know about you, but this verse surprises me a bit. We think of the towns of Sodom and Gomorrah as being full of sexual sin, but Ezekiel is clearly saying that Sodom was also guilty of pride, gluttony and laziness as well. The people were so self-absorbed that they were apathetic to the needs of the poor and needy right under their noses! If you have fear of lack, this can definitely cause you to want to hoard things (including food) for yourself and ignore those in need right in your own region. This is surely another reason why Isaiah 58 instructs us to share our food with the hungry when we are fasting. If this is speaking to you, then recognize it as an open door to the enemy to keep you in bondage to fear of lack. Ask the Lord to forgive you for not totally trusting and depending on Him for what you need to sustain your life. Ask Him to visit those times in your life where fear of lack came in and ask Him to shut those doors by the power of The Holy Spirit and the Blood of Jesus.

You may be asking yourself, "How can I pray a prayer asking the Lord to go back and touch areas that have already occurred?" We have to understand that God is not in time. We operate in time because He created the world to function using a system of hours, days, seasons, and so on. He can go back in time to any place or situation that caused fear and remove that fear at its root. Second Peter gives us a small glimpse of time by God's perspective:

2 Peter 3:8 (NLT) "But you must not forget this one thing, dear friends: A day is like a thousand years to the Lord, and a thousand years is like a day."

Remember Rachel in our last chapter? Here is her testimony of prayer utilizing this concept, that helped her greatly in her battle against eating disorders:

I started seeing Donna for counseling to help me overcome my eating disorder. I had struggled with anorexia, bulimia, over exercising, and over eating. One day I went to see

Donna for counseling. She asked me to go back in my mind and try to remember the first time I displayed symptoms of an eating disorder. I remembered a time when I was in second grade. I woke up on a Saturday morning to find no breakfast. My mother struggled with depression and frequently slept late. I ate an entire bag of Doritos, peanut butter rolled in powdered sugar, and pop-tarts smothered in butter. I started to feel sick. I didn't have to make myself throw up. My body just couldn't process all of the junk I had eaten and I got sick and threw up. Donna explained to me that The Holy Spirit could go back in time and heal me of my past. On my way home, I prayed in my car that The Holy Spirit would go back in time to that morning and stop me from eating that garbage. In the spirit, I spoke to little Rachel and told her to go upstairs and wake mommy up so she could make me breakfast. I could see the small, adorable version of myself look at me and say, "But mommy is too tired to make me breakfast." Just then, I saw Jesus standing next to little Rachel. He looked at her and said, "I will make you breakfast". I could see Jesus put a plate of food in front of little Rachel. The plate contained eggs, toast, and hash browns. I cried in my car as I could feel the healing from my past catching up to my present. After that moment in my car with the Lord, I went in my house. No one was home. It smelled like eggs, toast and hash browns in my apartment! The smell of breakfast was quite strong. It smelled as if someone was standing in my kitchen cooking right that very minute. I called my husband and asked him if he had cooked anything. He had no time to make breakfast before work and had only made a protein shake. No one had cooked the day before either as we ate leftovers. I dropped to my knees and cried thanking Jesus. I knew that he had prepared that meal for me in my past and he was showing me that the course of the past in my life had shifted. I learned that we can do this any time. We can ask the Holy Spirit to move through time and change things. If we are healed in our past, we are healed in the present. I'm so grateful as believers, we possess this supernatural, life changing tool! I am forever changed because God brought inner healing through His supernatural love.

Rachel

Isn't that amazing and awesome! Mistakes, traumatic events from your past and other sin induced fears and hurts can be removed with the precious Blood of Jesus and the power of The Holy Spirit. Those memories will no longer have unhealthy emotions tied to them. You must acknowledge that the same resurrection power that raised Jesus Christ from the dead is activated and available as a tool for your healing from the past. You are a three part being. You are physical body, soul, and spirit. Your spirit is regenerated when you accept Jesus into your heart/life to be your Lord and Savior. You still have issues in your soul and your body. If this were not the case, the minute you got saved, you would be made perfectly whole and healed in all areas of your life.

What other possible reasons do you overeat? Maybe you overeat not out of fear of lack, but a fear of loss of control. Fear of loss of control often follows sexual assault or molestation. I have seen many people build a wall of additional weight as a defense mechanism. If this applies to you, maybe you don't ever want to be touched in a sexual way again. Walls are built up around you because of fear and can be a conscious or sub-conscious way of keeping others at a distance. Putting on excess weight is an act of controlling who will come near you. God created you to be an interdependent being. If you starve yourself from relationships out of fear, you cause yourself to seek food (or other things) to fill the empty spaces where a healthy relationship could be growing and fulfilling your needs.

Anorexia and bulimia also can be rooted in fear of loss of control. Eating disorders are often birthed out of lack of control and un-forgiveness. If you suffer with an eating disorder, are you punishing yourself because you cannot control others' behavior? Maybe you haven't forgiven them. The unforgiveness causes unrest in your soul. You attempt to control the uneasiness by punishing your own body by starving or binging and purging. Anorexia seems to be rooted more in self unforgiveness and self destruction. Bulimia seems to be rooted more in unforgiveness of others. If you are suffering with either of these eating disorders, I urge you to seek Christian counseling.

Make peace with the ones you have not forgiven. Speak forgiveness out loud over and over again as an act of obedience to the Lord. Your heart will eventually catch up with what your mouth is speaking. Unforgiveness is toxic to your mind, body, emotions, etc. I have included a prayer of forgiveness to help guide you through the path to freedom:

PRAYER OF FORGIVENESS

Father God, I come to You through the Blood of the Lamb. You know my heart has pent up unforgiveness that tortures and defiles me. I come to You now asking for Your divine help in releasing that unforgiveness. Of myself I can do nothing. Without You, I am nothing.

I lay _____ on the altar of forgiveness and ask You, Holy Father, to pour down Your cleansing fire on our relationship. I sacrifice my rights I feel that are mine to hold myself and _____ in bondage to the unforgiveness.

With Your power, Lord, I completely and totally forgive_____
for any wrong-doing that has caused me pain.

I now pray that You pour out Your richest blessings upon_____.
Allow us both to feel the shift in the spiritual atmosphere as forgiveness sets the captives free.

In Jesus' name I pray, Amen.

Remember in prior chapters you read how unforgiveness causes you to judge, criticize, and then run to food for comfort? Meditate on what was conveyed in the book of James:

James 3:2 (NLT) " Indeed, we all make many mistakes. For if we could control our tongues, we would be perfect and could also control ourselves in every other way."

What a glorious thought to be able to control ourselves in every way, if only we could control our tongues. Walking in forgiveness will assist you in controlling the words you speak because your record of wrongs will be cleared with others. Can you see how important the tongue is even in gluttony?

What else is an open door to gluttony? How about entitlement? Do you feel as though you deserve to overeat? Do you use it as a way of self-medicating with sugar or comfort food? Do you reward yourself with food for a job well done? Spend some time with God and ask Him to show you how this may apply to your eating habits. Meditate on this Psalm and write down some ways that you can reward yourself without food.

Psalm 34:8 (NLT) "Oh, taste and see that the Lord is good! Blessed is the man who takes refuge in him!"

As you choose to walk away from the sin of gluttony, pray this prayer with a sincere heart:

Forgive me, Lord, for reaching for food out of a sense of entitlement, unforgiveness or a need to control, or out of fear of lack. I don't have any right to eat more than my body needs. I thank You that You are providing what I do need and thank You for renewing my mind in this area.

Believe that the Lord can do this for you. Meditate on His power and might. Soak into your spirit that the Lord has no equal.

Isaiah 40:25-31 <u>New Living Translation </u>(NLT)

25 "To whom will you compare Me? Who is My equal?" asks the Holy One.

26 Look up into the heavens. Who created all the stars? He brings them out like an army, one after another, calling each by its name. Because of his great power and incomparable strength, not a single one is missing. 27 O Jacob, how can you say the Lord does not see your troubles? O Israel, how can you say God ignores your rights? 28 Have you never heard? Have you never understood? The Lord is the everlasting God, the Creator of all the earth. He never grows weak or weary. No one can measure the depths of His understanding. 29 He gives power to the weak and strength to the powerless. 30 Even youths will become weak and tired, and young men will fall in exhaustion. 31 But those who trust in the Lord will find new strength. They will soar high on wings like eagles. They will run and not grow weary. They will walk and not faint."

God has everything you need to escape these places in your mind and in your heart.

Isaiah 41:13 (NLT) "For I hold you by your right hand - I, the Lord your God. And I say to you,'Don't be afraid. I am here to help you."

Wow! Thank God every day that He declares He is here to help you!

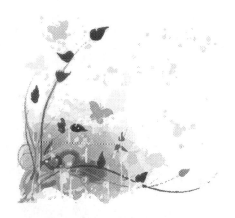

Notes

Chapter 6

Perfectionism

In this chapter I am most often referencing the Amplified version of God's Word. I felt this version would best represent the insights I am making regarding perfectionism.

The definition of perfectionism is *a demand of excellence and rejection of anything less than perfect.* Do you demand excellence from yourself and others? Do you reject anything that is less than your idea of perfection?

Perfectionism can also be considered a personality trait characterized by a person's striving for flawlessness and setting excessively high performance standards. Often you may become overly critical of yourself and expect high levels of performance from yourself regardless of what is happening in your life. When others criticize you it may be absolutely crushing to your self-esteem. Maybe you set unattainable goals and then punish yourself with negative words if you don't reach these goals. Perfectionism is a cruel taskmaster.

Take a few minutes and jot down the answers to these questions when it comes to your body image and perfectionism. Who's standard are you reaching for? Is it God's? What or who are you comparing yourself to? What is your measuring stick for perfection regarding what you think your body should look like? Is it the world's idea of how your body should look? Are you comparing yourself to others?

Comparison is another way of saying "I envy your body type" or "I would love to be aging as gracefully as so and so." It says, "I must attain the standard and find a way to maintain it, even if it is not how God made me."

This type of striving for perfection is a form of jealousy. Let's take a look in God's Word and see what jealousy can do to you.

Proverbs 27:4 (AMPC) says, *"Wrath is cruel and anger is an overwhelming flood, but who is able to stand before jealousy?"*

You can see in *Proverbs 14:30 (NLT) "A peaceful heart leads to a healthy body; jealousy is like cancer in the bones."*

Ecclesiastes 4:4 (NLT) "Then I observed that most people are motivated to success because they envy their neighbors. But this, too is meaningless - like chasing the wind."

How does perfectionism, driven by jealousy, affect you? The Sadducees and Pharisees were filled with a jealousy of Jesus' ministry and His Apostles as they preached the Gospel and displayed miracles, signs, and wonders. Probe deeper and you'll see that many times jealousy and envy compel you to perfectionism and can be tied to having a religious spirit. You compare and judge others. In this case you are comparing yourself to others and striving for what may be unattainable.

If you strive for perfection in your body image, you may have had times of success. Most of you can *white knuckle* it through a time period of what you think of as perfection on your own. During this time of triumph, pride can set in. You think you have this whole diet, exercise lifestyle down to a science and your way is the right way. During this time with the door cracked open by pride, you may be judging others based on what you see them eat. You may silently (or not so silently) judge them for their lack of exercise and/or lack of knowledge about eating the way you do. You start to think of certain foods as poisonous and others as holy. Let's read what Jesus said in Matthew:

Matthew 15:16-18 (AMPC) "16 And He said, Are you also even yet dull and ignorant [without understanding and [a]unable to put things together]? 17 Do you not see and understand that whatever goes into the mouth passes into the [b]abdomen and so passes on into the place where discharges are deposited?18 But whatever comes out of the mouth comes from the heart, and this is what makes a man unclean and defiles [him]."

It's a slippery slope. You start to analyze everything and label foods as good or bad. You begin to worry about eating something you have labeled as bad. How does God respond to your worry and perfectionism regarding what you eat?

Philippians 4:6 (AMPC) says, " Do not fret or have any anxiety about anything, but in every circumstance and in everything, by prayer and petition ([a]definite requests), with thanksgiving, continue to make your wants known to God."

Meditate on this Scripture as it would pertain to your eating and exercise.

How about when you are casting judgmental eyes at someone not eating the way you do?

Romans 2:1 (AMPC) says, "Therefore you have no excuse or defense or justification, O man, whoever you are who judges and condemns another. For in posing as judge and passing sentence on another, you condemn yourself, because you who judge are habitually practicing the very same things [that you censure and denounce]."

Document what the Lord is saying to you about judgement.

Can you take a moment and examine your motives for wanting a better body? Measure your motives against this scripture in the book of James:

James 4:2-3 (AMPC) "2 You are jealous and covet [what others have] and your desires go unfulfilled; [so] you become murderers. [To hate is to murder as far as your hearts are concerned.] You burn with envy and anger and are not able to obtain [the gratification, the contentment, and the happiness that you seek], so you fight and war. You do not have, because you do not ask.3 [Or] you do ask [God for them] and yet fail to receive, because you ask with wrong purpose and evil, selfish motives. Your intention is [when you get what you desire] to spend it in sensual pleasures."

What are your motives? Do you want to have a great body for your own satisfaction when you look in the mirror or see a certain number when you step on the scale? Do you want to do lose weight in an unhealthy, unbalanced way because it is quick or painless, requiring less willpower on your behalf. Is it the latest diet or scientific research that tells you to avoid fat, carbs, salt, meat, wheat or whatever that seems to be the surest way to permanent success? Most people struggling with their weight and body image have fallen into some quick fix eating plan at least once in their lives.

Perfectionism can be a great measuring stick to show you how much agreement you have with the world.

James 4:4-6(AMPC) 4 "You [are like] unfaithful wives [having illicit love affairs with the world and breaking your marriage vow to God]! Do you not know that being the world's friend is being God's enemy? So whoever chooses to be a friend of the world takes his stand as an enemy of God.5 Or do you suppose that the Scripture is speaking to no purpose that says, The Spirit Whom He has caused to dwell in us yearns over us and He yearns for the Spirit [to be welcome] with a jealous love?6 But He gives us more and more grace ([a]power of the Holy Spirit, to meet this evil tendency and all others fully). That is why He says, God sets Himself against the proud and haughty, but gives grace [continually] to the lowly (those who are humble enough to receive it)."

If you have been praying the prayers in the previous chapters, you have been breaking friendship with the world and humbling yourself under the mighty hand of God.

As you humble yourself, it's easier to practice James 4:7-8 (NLT) which says, *"So humble yourselves before God. Resist the devil and he will flee from you and He will come close to you."* 8 *"Come close to God and He will come close to you. "Wash your hands, you sinners; and purify your hearts, for your loyalty is divided between God and the world."* As you purify your heart, your loyalty will no longer be divided between God and the world. Verse 9 gives you permission to be sad about the way you have treated your body, judged others and rejected yourself. *James 4:9 (NLT) "Let there be tears for what you have done. Let there be sorrow and deep grief. Let there be sadness instead of laughter, and gloom instead of joy."* This verse leads to Godly repentance. *This repentance opens your heart to change.* This is the humbling that comes in verse 10 where it is written, *"Humble yourselves before the Lord and He will lift you up in honor."* God will do the lifting for you.

Does the thought of God doing the work of lifting you up make you feel anxious or out of control? Do you feel like there must be some other piece of the puzzle that is your responsibility? You may be dealing with more striving and perfectionism than you realized when you started to read this chapter. Just because you don't look perfect and your house and children aren't perfect doesn't mean you don't wrestle with perfectionism.

Consider the Proverbs 31 woman. She can be overwhelming and many men and women have written about her. Some believe that this woman is actually many different women while others will put you under a yoke of bondage and say her entire job description must be done daily to be of worth to God, your husband, and your children. Clear your slate of all of these possibilities and come away with me to your daily prayer time with the Lord (whatever amount of time you have).

I am going to share a concept of surrender that will bring more peace to your days. Take note paper and pen with you for your time with God. As you open in prayer ask the Holy Spirit to only bring to your mind (during your prayer time) the tasks that He wants you to accomplish today. Don't write down what YOU want to do that day, but only what tasks come to mind as you are going through your time of prayer.

Jot each down on the note paper as they come up and then immediately get back to prayer. As you finish your prayer time and look at your list. Be sure to do only the things on the list for that day.

Can you see how having God set the agenda for your day will free you up from self-guilt or any other voices of condemnation that say you didn't accomplish enough today? This method is divine. I know a woman who avoided a robbery by not going to the bank until God allowed it in her routine one day. Another person reported visiting people in the hospital and making more time in their routine for others. This was not something they would normally take the time to do. One friend who practices this technique, got her daily list done just before the school called for her to pick up sick children. When your daily agenda is the Lord's, you will feel accomplished and fulfilled.

You may be asking what this has to do with eating and weight loss, etc. When you are walking in God's divine order for your day, you will feel less stress, less guilt, less expectation of others, etc. These are the unhealthy emotions that can cause you to overeat for comfort or to stuff down an accusing voice that you are trying to silence. For many people that accusing voice says, "You did not accomplish enough today, therefore you aren't worth very much to anyone." If this speaks to you, I am guessing that you are exhausted from trying to reach the elusive state of perfection. If you are tired of all the negative self-talk and/or running in circles (that God never intended for your day), you may tend to reach for sugar or caffeine to counteract the exhaustion. You are not alone. Why do you think that coffee houses and bakeries are all the rage right now? People are pumping themselves full of caffeine and sugar to keep up with the demands imposed upon them.

Let's get back to Proverbs 31. As you read below, ask the Holy Spirit to illuminate how His order for each day fulfills the call of duty as an excellent wife/woman. If you are a man reading this chapter, I invite you to read Proverbs 31 in view of you being the bride of Christ.

Proverbs 31:10-31 (AMPC) "10 A capable, intelligent, and [a] virtuous woman—who is he who can find her? She is far more precious than jewels and her value is far above rubies or pearls. 11 The heart of her husband trusts in her confidently and relies on and believes in her securely, so that he has no lack of [honest] gain or need of [dishonest]spoil. 12 She comforts, encourages, and does him only good as long as there is life within her.13 She seeks out wool and flax and works with willing hands [to develop it]. 14 She is like the merchant ships loaded with foodstuffs; she brings her household's food from a far [country].15 She rises while it is yet night and gets [spiritual] food for her household and assigns her maids their tasks. 16 She considers a [new] field before she buys or accepts it [expanding prudently and not courting neglect of her present duties by assuming other duties]; with her savings [of time and strength] she plants fruitful vines in her vineyard.17 She girds herself with strength [spiritual, mental, and physical fitness for her God-given task] and makes her arms strong and firm. 18 She tastes and sees that her gain from work [with and for God] is good; her lamp goes not out, but it burns on continually through the night [of trouble, privation, or sorrow, warning away fear, doubt, and distrust]. 19 She lays her hands to the spindle, and her hands hold the distaff. 20 She opens her hand to the poor, yes, she reaches out her filled hands to the needy [whether in body, mind, or spirit]. 21 She fears not the snow for her family, for all her household are doubly clothed in scarlet. 22 She makes for herself coverlets, cushions, and rugs of tapestry. Her clothing is of linen, pure and fine, and of purple [such as that of which the clothing of the priests and the hallowed cloths of the temple were made]. 23 Her husband is known in the [city's] gates, when he sits among the elders of the land. 24 She makes fine linen garments and leads others to buy them; she delivers to the merchants girdles [or sashes that free one up for service]. 25 Strength and dignity are her clothing and her position is strong and secure; she rejoices over the future [the latter day or time to come, knowing that she and her family are in readiness for it]! 26 She opens her mouth in skillful and godly wisdom, and on her tongue is the law of kindness [giving counsel and instruction]. 27 She looks well to how things go in her household, and the bread of idleness (gossip, discontent, and self-pity) she will not eat. 28 Her children rise up and call her blessed (happy, fortunate, and to be envied); and her husband boasts of and praises her, [saying], 29 [b]Many daughters have done virtuously, nobly, and well [with the strength of character that is steadfast in goodness], but you excel them all. 30 Charm and grace are deceptive, and beauty is vain [because it is not lasting], but a woman who reverently and worshipfully fears the Lord, she shall be praised! 31 Give her of the fruit of her hands, and let her own works praise her in the gates [of the city]!"

Take a look at the footnotes from biblegateway.com. They should help you glean even more insight as to what God is saying to you right now. **Footnotes: as written from biblegateway.com:**

a. <u>Proverbs 31:10</u> It is most unfortunate that this description of God's ideal woman is usually confined in readers' minds merely to its literal sense—her ability as a homemaker, as in the picture of Martha of Bethany in Luke 10:38-42. But it is obvious that far more than that is meant. When the summary of what makes her value "far above rubies" is given (in Prov. 31:30), it is her spiritual life only that is mentioned. One can almost hear the voice of Jesus saying, "Mary has chosen the good portion... which shall not be taken away from her" (Luke 10:42).

b. Proverbs 31:29 "Many daughters have done... nobly and well... but you excel them all." What a glowing description here recorded of this woman in private life, this "capable, intelligent, and virtuous woman" of Prov. 31! It means she had done more than Miriam, the one who led a nation's women in praise to God (Exod. 15:20, 21); Deborah, the patriotic military advisor (Judg. 4:4-10); Ruth, the woman of constancy (Ruth 1:16); Hannah, the ideal mother (I Sam. 1:20; 2:19); the Shunammite, the hospitable woman (II Kings 4:8-10); Huldah, the woman who revealed God's secret message to national leaders (II Kings 22:14); and even more than Queen Esther, the woman who risked sacrificing her life for her people (Esth. 4:16). In what way did she "excel them all"? In her spiritual and practical devotion to God, which permeated every area and relationship of her life. All seven of the Christian virtues (II Pet. 1:5) are there, like colored threads in a tapestry. Her secret, which is open to everyone, is the Holy Spirit's climax to the story, and to this book. In Prov. 31:30, it becomes clear that the "reverent *and* worshipful fear of the Lord," which is "the beginning (the chief and choice part) of Wisdom" (Prov. 9:10), is put forth as the true foundation for a life which is valued by God and her husband as "far above rubies *or* pearls" (Prov. 31:10).

Dear heavenly Father, thank You for the value You have placed on my life. Forgive me for striving toward perfectionism. I ask You to guide me daily to walk in Your agenda for my household. I choose to lay aside my ideas and choose Your peace and Your order each day. In Jesus' name I pray, Amen.

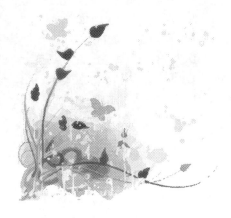

Notes

Chapter 7

Lust of the flesh, Lust of the eyes, Pride of life and Jonah revisited

Most of you are very familiar with the account of how Jesus was led into the wilderness after he was baptized. Matthew clearly tells us what happened next:

Matthew 4:1-11 (NLT) 4 "Then Jesus was led by the Spirit into the wilderness to be tempted there by the devil. 2 For forty days and forty nights he fasted and became very hungry. 3 During that time the devil[a] came and said to him, "If you are the Son of God, tell these stones to become loaves of bread."4 But Jesus told him, "No! The Scriptures say,'People do not live by bread alone, but by every word that comes from the mouth of God.'[b]"5 Then the devil took him to the holy city, Jerusalem, to the highest point of the Temple, 6 and said, "If you are the Son of God, jump off! For the Scriptures say,'He will order his angels to protect you. And they will hold you up with their hands so you won't even hurt your foot on a stone.'[c]"7 Jesus responded, "The Scriptures also say, 'You must not test the Lord your God.'[d]"8 Next the devil took him to the peak of a very high mountain and showed him all the kingdoms of the world and their glory. 9 "I will give it all to you," he said, "if you will kneel down and worship me." 10 "Get out of here, Satan," Jesus told him. "For the Scriptures say,'You must worship the Lord your God and serve only Him.'[e]" 11 Then the devil went away, and angels came and took care of Jesus."

Let's begin with *lust of the flesh. Flesh* can speak of your actual body or it can be a reference to things that oppose what the Spirit of God is desiring us to do. When Jesus spoke to the devil, regarding *flesh* (verse 4,) He was quoting:

Deuteronomy 8:3 (AMP)3 "And He humbled you and allowed you to hunger and fed you with manna, which you did not know nor did your fathers know, that He might make you recognize and personally know that man does not live by bread only, but man lives by every word that proceeds out of the mouth of the Lord."

I am trusting that you, as a spirit filled believer, have experienced times of being filled to overflowing with the Holy Ghost. When that occurs, have you noticed that during those times, you aren't as hungry or have virtually no appetite at all? When you are in His holy presence, you are being sustained, satiated, and upheld by the Spirit of God. Your flesh doesn't desire food in the same way when your focus is on Him.

When the focus is on food, you are most likely focusing on self and you feel out of control. This lack of control should be a clear indicator that you need to soak in His presence. How do you do that? Spend time praying in your prayer language or you can make time to close your eyes and listen to worship music that focuses on Him and His majesty. If all you have is five minutes, stand still and just focus on Jesus. Praise His

Holy name! The Bible says that the Lord inhabits our praises. As you praise, you will feel His presence and peace. He has everything you will ever need.

Next, I want you to focus on *lust of the eyes*. The NLT Bible refers to this as *a craving for everything you see*. This conjures up for me a vision of a buffet filled with all different types of foods. From one end of the steam tables to as far as the eye can see, are savory items of all different ethnic origins. Oh, and you can't forget the sweets! Rows of cakes, puddings, cookies and an ice cream station spanning out into the distance are available at this food fest! Would your old nature be able to stand up against such a worthy foe? Before the Lord broke these bondages over me, I would not have stood a chance! I am not a fan of buffets, but if I have to meet friends or family in such an establishment, I allow the Holy Spirit to help me make my choices and I stop eating when I'm comfortable. What others are choosing to eat has no power over me.

Remember what a stumbling block cravings were for Eve? She saw that the fruit of the tree was very desirable. She may have even wondered if it tasted superior to the other fruit on the other trees. As with most things belonging to this world, the deceptive fruit only led to death and destruction. Isn't it like that at a buffet? Many times the food looks very appetizing, however, when you actually taste it, it's barely worth the calories that you just swallowed! Don't allow the allure of tempting food to override the Holy Spirit's leading as you walk in your new found freedom.

As you look at the *pride of life* as it pertains to this study, you see the NLT Bible describes it as *pride in your achievements and possessions*. It's important that your new goals regarding body image do not become your newest idol. Don't put yourself back under subjection to *possessing or achieving* a certain physical appearance. You want to take care of yourself and put your best out there for people to see, but not to the point of idolatry. Make a commitment to yourself to have no expectations regarding the outcome of this journey with the Lord. Allow Him to slowly, gently take you where He desires to lead you with your weight and your physical appearance.

As we began Chapter 1, you were reminded that Jonah had to be in the belly of a whale in order to face all he needed to see about his own fears and disobedience. As we close, let's revisit Jonah in Chapter 2.

Jonah 2:2 (NLT) He said, "I cried out to the Lord in my great trouble, and He answered me. I called to You from the land of the dead, and Lord, You heard me!"

When you cry, He hears you. When you have tried everything the world has to offer and you are in the belly of the whale (Sheol), He hears. Jonah 2:6 says, *"He brings our lives up from the pit."*

Jonah 2:7-10 (NLT) 7 "As my life was slipping away, I remembered the Lord. And my earnest prayer went out to You in Your holy Temple. 8 Those who worship false gods turn their backs on all God's mercies. 9 But I will offer sacrifices to You with songs of praise, and I will fulfill all my vows. For my salvation comes from the Lord alone." 10 Then the Lord ordered the fish to spit Jonah out onto the beach."

Notice as Jonah focuses on the Lord with remembrance, prayer, repentance of false gods, and finally with praises, he is delivered! Obedience brings revelation. Obedience *with* the revelation, brings breakthrough, blessing, and instruction for moving forward.

When you aren't bowing down before the false gods that consume your thoughts, you hear God more clearly. Shut down the distractions. What are your distractions? Were they the old issues that you prayed through in the previous chapters? If so, you are free from all of those things that the Holy Spirit has assisted you in rooting out. Stay out of that old pit! If you are still distracted by some worldly snares, you may need to fast them for a season, if not permanently. Two things I had to fast for a season in this journey were women's magazines and cooking shows. Most women's magazines have a carefully planned agenda. They are designed to take you from wanting to look like the clothing models in the first part of the magazine to comparing yourself to them. Next, about midway through the magazine, are some sort of diet and the healthy eating tips du jour. Most magazines end with fattening recipes. It can be quite the emotional roller coaster from cover to cover. Magazines no longer cause me to stumble because now I understand the trap. Cooking shows really caused me to want to eat even when I wasn't really hungry. Regarding watching cooking shows, I have decided to make it an occasional past time. I love gleaning ideas but must monitor how much I can view before it becomes a potential old trap.

Let's break down verses 7-10 in Jonah, chapter 2. Verse seven says that when your soul faints is when you earnestly and sincerely remember the Lord. I really appreciate that God allows you the freedom to get to the end of yourself so that the only place you can turn is to Him. He is so gracious to you and uses those moments to remind you that He is the ONE with all the answers!

Verse eight reminds you that paying regard to useless and worthless idols causes you to forsake your own source of mercy and loving kindness. Take a moment and ask the Lord if you have any other idols or stumbling blocks (like my magazines and T.V. shows) that could cause you to stay out of victory. What are your idols? Name them out loud. If He shows you an area, ask for forgiveness and fast your stumbling block. God may allow you to add it back into your life at some point, or He may not. I am okay with magazines now because I understand the trap; however, I can only occasionally watch cooking shows on television. It used to be a daily occurrence for me and now it is more like a bi-monthly event.

Verse nine says you are to offer your voice up in thanksgiving because salvation and deliverance belong to the Lord. Thank the Lord often for delivering you from the snare of food bondage. He deserves all the glory, honor, and praise.

Notice then in verse ten that when Jonah took responsibility for his rebellion and put focus on the Lord, then God told the fish to spit him back on dry land. His heart was right and Jonah could now be used by the Lord. It is all about getting your heart right with God. As you meditate on your responsibility for how you got to this place (not in condemnation, but sincerity of heart), earnestly seek and remember (think on) the Lord. I believe your prayer will be heard by Him in His holy temple.

Ask yourself this sobering question. How can you allow God to use you in a full capacity when you are self-conscious about the way you look and feel about yourself? There is so much freedom in not having your whole day focused on what you are and are not eating or carrying guilt because you didn't exercise.

Whether you are bothered by five pounds or two hundred five pounds, the thoughts that trouble you and interfere with your day are basically the same. If you have a lot of weight to lose, your journey will take a bit longer, but if you don't take responsibility, it will continue to rob you of joy, health, and the fulfillment of your destiny.

The way you feel about yourself can greatly veer you off the track that God wants you on in order to fulfill your destiny. Take it one day at a time and follow His leading.

Remember when the whale spit Jonah out he was put miraculously right back on the mediterranean coast. God made sure that Jonah was positioned to complete his task. Delivering the message to Nineveh was part of Jonah fulfilling his destiny. God has a destiny for you and He will get you back on the track from which you veered off, just as He did for Jonah.

It's time to take back the territory that the enemy has stolen from you. You don't stand still as a human being. You are either gaining or losing territory. I believe if you have prayed the prayers in the previous chapters, you have gained much territory! Don't look at the mountain in front of you. Look at your Savior and take it one meal at a time, one step at a time. He is able to do exceedingly, abundantly above anything you could ask or think!

Dear Heavenly Father, I thank you for taking me through this journey of self-discovery and acceptance. You are truly my Rock, my Healer and my Deliverer! You are always faithful to surround me with your goodness and your love!

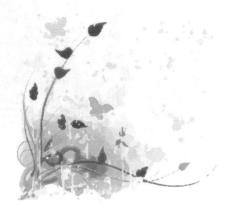

Notes

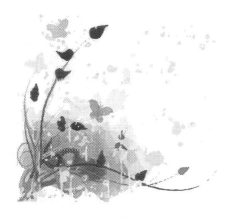

Afterword

As the writing portion of this project came to a close, God spoke a word into me. He said that *if I would begin to run for exercise 3 times per week, he would heal my physical body.* That was two years ago and my running journey has indeed brought increased strength and healing to my feet, ankles, knees, hips and back! Within the first six months of running, God called me to begin blogging about the revelations He was giving me as I would run. I invite you to follow my ongoing journey at www.revelationsontherun.com.

When I first began this project, I thought it would be mainly for men and women who are struggling with typical food issues. As more people have field tested this book, we are experiencing the joy of seeing those suffering with anorexia and bulimia set free as well. I couldn't be happier! If you know someone who struggles with either eating disorder (or both), please bless them with a copy. You may save their life! Visit our newest blog site where great discussions are happening on Anorexia, Bulimia, exercise and food in general. Even though this web site is geared toward Christians looking for God's answers to eating disorders, I pray it will be a beacon of light and hope to all.

www.anaannabelle.com

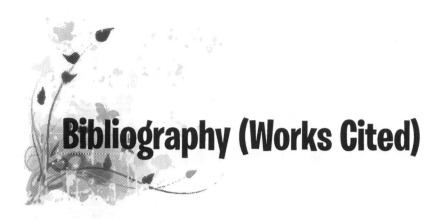

Bibliography (Works Cited)

You Are Not What You Weigh - by Lisa Bevere
Copyright 1998 Published by Siloam, Lake Mary, FL

The Oxford English Dictionary
Oxford University Press, Oxford, NY
copyright 2000

www.yourdictionary.com

Footnotes: www.biblegateway.com

Printed in the United States
By Bookmasters